DELTA DIET™

GEORGE E. ABRAHAM II, MD

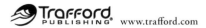 www.trafford.com

North America & international
toll-free: 1 888 232 4444 (USA & Canada)
phone: 250 383 6864 ♦ fax: 812 355 4082

Contents

Abstract – Delta Diet™

The Delta Diet is a weight management program based on utilizing natural daily body hormone cycles (Circadian cycle) to achieve and maintain a desirable body weight. This program enables moderately overweight people to achieve and maintain an ideal body weight range without resorting to medications, surgery, or other drastic measures. The program is based on the triad of HORMONES, NUTRIENT TIMING, and the CIRCADIAN SLEEP-WAKE CYCLE. If implemented faithfully, this program will usually produce results in a few weeks to a few months, and the results can be maintained indefinitely.

I.

Introduction – Delta Diet™

The word Circadian refers to a rhythm based on a 24-hour period of time. Another word commonly used for this type of periodic rhythm is Diurnal. The term Circadian Rhythm refers to a daily rhythmic activity cycle based on a 24-hour rhythm. What's so important about that? Simply, many living organisms, including humans, have adapted themselves, over millennia, to a 24-hour life cycle that corresponds to the rate of rotation of the earth on its axis. All the hormones that control our metabolism fluctuate according to a 24-hour cycle. Understanding these hormone cycles holds an important key to good health, including weight control.

This book will explain how our daily hormone fluctuations control metabolism, and how the knowledge of these fluctuations can be used to advantage to achieve and maintain a healthy weight, while at the same time promoting good health in general. Application of the principles presented here will help a motivated person to achieve their goal of normal weight and good health on a long-term basis.

I I

What Can We Learn From The Bear?

Hibernation is a sleep-like state that some animals go into during winter, protecting them from the cold and reducing their need for food at a time when food is scarce. Animals that hibernate consume large amounts of food in the autumn to prepare for hibernation. This food is stored as fat in their bodies, and used as food (fuel for metabolism) during the long hibernation. These animals also lower their metabolism during hibernation, reducing their need for food and ensuring that the supply of stored fat is adequate.

Bears are not true hibernators, because their metabolism doesn't decrease much during their winter sleep, and they "burn up" much, if not all, of the fat they store before winter. If bears did not use most of their fat during the winter hibernation, I wonder how "obese" they would be? I also wonder how much fat humans "burn" during their brief daily sleep, averaging 6 to 8 hours?

It turns out that this concept of fat storage during periods of inactivity, especially during the sleep portion of our daily (diurnal) Circadian cycle, is extremely important in understanding why many people are overweight, and also in understanding how weight can be controlled and managed.

III.

The Hormones

Hormones are chemical messengers that are produced by the numerous glands of the endocrine system. Hormones circulate in the bloodstream and control the functioning of the various cells of the body. A good example is thyroid hormone, which controls the rate at which the cells produce energy by combining oxygen and nutrients, similar to the "idle" on an automobile engine. If the "idle" is set too low, the engine becomes sluggish and inefficient and may stall. If the "idle" is set too high, the engine overheats. The body responds to too little or too much thyroid hormone in the same way. Too little, and it becomes sluggish; too much, and it "overheats", producing bad effects on the heart (rapid heart beat) and breaking down fat and protein in an unhealthy way.

The hormones that cycle on a daily basis (Circadian rhythm) are the corticosteroids (cortisol being the main player), and epinephrine (adrenalin). These substances are produced in the adrenal glands, and play important roles in the sleep-wake cycle.

They also have significant effects on the way nutrients are used by the body, either burned as fuel by the "working" cells, or stored as fat in fat cells. There are numerous other hormones important to bodily functioning, but their levels in the blood do not exhibit the Circadian rhythm, and will not be discussed here.

For people on a normal sleep-wake cycle, the levels of epinephrine and cortisol in the blood tend to peak at about 8:00AM daily, and reach their lowest point in the late afternoon or early evening, as shown in Figure 1.

FIGURE 1

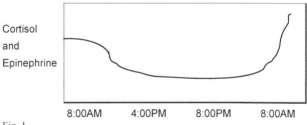

Fig. 1

An area of the brain called the hypothalamus controls this daily cycling of hormones and its relation to the sleep-wake cycle. The higher hormone levels in the morning prepare the body for wakening and subsequent daily activities, while the lower levels in the evening prepare the body for sleep. Because of the effect of these hormones on the body metabolism, calories are consumed at a higher rate during the "wake" portion of the cycle, and at a lower rate during the "sleep" portion. If too many calories are consumed at the evening meal, particularly from foods that are easily broken down into glucose quickly (high glycemic index foods such as sugar, white flour products, white rice, white potatoes, etc.), these excess calories are likely to be stored as fat during the relative inactivity of sleep (a brief period of hibernation), while calories consumed in the morning are likely to be used immediately for energy production to do physical work BEFORE they can be converted to fat. This concept is the basis for Circadian weight management and the Delta Diet program.

IV.

Why Three Meals A Day?

Have you ever wondered why humans usually eat three meals a day? The answer is that most likely we have adapted to our environment by evolution over time. As our bodies evolved in order to best survive in our environment, the mechanisms for providing nutrients (energy) also evolved. Our intestinal tract is "designed" by evolution, for what engineers call "batch processing" (batch feeding). When we eat a meal, the food is initially held and processed (digested) in the stomach for about 30 minutes to 1 hour, and then fed continuously into the small intestine, where the nutrients are further processed into their smallest components (simple sugars, fatty acids, amino acids, etc.). These components are then absorbed into the circulation over several hours time.

When the stomach is full, the perception of hunger decreases through a complex mechanism including a rise in blood glucose levels. When the stomach is empty, and when blood glucose levels fall, we perceive hunger. Based on the volume of food our stomachs can hold, our batch feedings (meals) provide about 4 to 6 hours of energy, which we use to do work, after which we begin to sense hunger. If we don't do enough physical work to "burn up" all the energy stored in the food we consume, the left-over food calories tend to be stored in the fat cells in the body for later use. Unfortunately, once fat is produced and stored, the body has difficulty breaking it down into its basic components that can be utilized for energy. The use of nutrients for energy immediately after they are consumed and before they can be stored as fat is much more efficient.

Hence, the TIMING of food intake in relation to our daily activities is critical in determining how the body will use the food (either burn immediately to provide energy to do work, or store as fat). Also, the proper timing of the nutritional components (carbohydrate, fat, and protein) is critical in terms of how they are utilized. For example, foods which are easily converted by the body to fat, such as those with a high glycemic index (sugar, white flour products, white rice, potatoes), should be eaten preferentially before periods of physical activity, such as at the beginning of the work day, rather than just prior to going to sleep.

V.

What Is Overweight And Why Is It Bad?

Body weight can be considered to be either healthy or unhealthy. Unhealthy body weight can be either too low or too high to maintain good health. The conditions that produce a body weight that is too low are called eating disorders. The condition which is manifested as a body weight which is excessive is called overweight, or in the extreme, obesity. Obesity can be considered a "fat storage" disease.

The overweight, or obese, condition (particularly "abdominal" obesity) has been shown to be an independent predictor of numerous poor health outcomes, including diseases of the heart and arteries, elevated blood glucose, insulin resistance, Type 2 diabetes mellitus, elevated blood lipids (cholesterol, triglycerides, free fatty acids), high blood pressure, increased tendency for blood clotting, strokes, gallstones, sleep apnea, and various cancers including breast, endometrial, and colon cancer. The more overweight the person is, the greater the risk that one or more of these conditions will develop, leading to a poor quality of life and premature death. Other by-products of the overweight condition include degenerative arthritis of the weight-bearing joints (low back, hips, knees, and ankles), and psychological factors related to the perceived unaesthetic appearance of the body both to the overweight person and to others.

Other than aesthetic appearance, how can you tell if you are overweight? Numerous methods to measure the overweight condition have been developed, and none are perfect. However, as a group, these measures can reasonably predict the degree of health risk associated with your weight. The most commonly used measures of overweight are the Body-Mass Index, the Percent Body-Fat, the Waist-to-Hip ratio, and the Waist Circumference, and these will now be described.

Body Mass Index (BMI) is a commonly use measure of overweight which relates weight to height, the premise being that taller people can weigh more and still be healthy, a premise which turns out, in fact, to be true.

$$BMI = Weight \ (kilograms)/Height \ (meters) \ squared$$

OR

$$BMI = 704.5 \ x \ Weight \ (pounds)/Height \ (feet) \ squared$$

Appendix 4 is a table which shows BMI in relation to height and weight. Figure 2 shows health risk in relation to BMI. A BMI between 18.5 and 25 equates to optimal health risk. A BMI less than 18.5 indicates undernutrition and increased health risk. A BMI between 25 and 30 is called OVERWEIGHT, indicating mildly increased health risk. A BMI of 30 or greater is called OBESITY, and indicates progressively increasing health risk.

The advantages of the BMI are that it is easy to measure and that it correlates well with health risk for people with average build (ratio of body fat to muscle). However, for people with high body muscle mass (low body fat), BMI is not as good a predictor of health risk.

The Percent Body Fat (percent of body weight which is fat), although a good marker for physical conditioning and low health risk, is technically difficult to measure and therefore not a practically useful index of health risk with regard to obesity.

The Waist Circumference is probably the most useful predictor of health risk related to overweight because it is easy to measure and provides a measure of abdominal fat, which, as noted above, is the best predictor of a number of serious health conditions. The Waist Circumference is measured at the level of the uppermost pelvic bones (iliac crest). A properly measured waist circumference greater than 35 inches in women and 40 inches in men indicates high health risk.

The Hip-to-Waist Ratio is similar to the Waist Circumference in that it is a measure of abdominal fat, but is harder to measure and is probably not as accurate in predicting health risk. The Waist Circumference is therefore recommended.

Since no one index or measure is perfect, a combination of indexes is preferable in trying to assess health risk. The best combination that can be recommended at this time appears to be BMI and Waist Circumference.

FIGURE 2

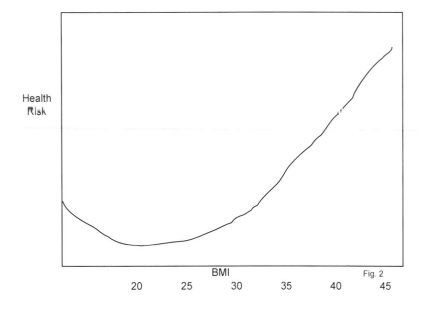

Health Risk

BMI

Fig. 2

20   25   30   35   40   45

VI

Food - Our Energy Source

The primary components of food are the energy-providing nutrients (carbohydrates, fats, and proteins), vitamins, minerals, fiber, and water.

1. CARBOHYDRATES: (Remember, all carbohydrates are not created equal).

Carbohydrates (Carbs) in the diet consist of simple carbohydrates (disaccharides such as sucrose, which is table sugar) and complex carbohydrates. Complex carbs include starches which come primarily from potatoes and processed grains such as rice and white flour products, and are easily digested into simple carbs, and what are called structural carbs, which are not completely digestible and are a good source of fiber (these include fruits, vegetables, and whole grains, especially when uncooked). Simple carbs and starches are digested in the small intestine into glucose, which is then absorbed into the bloodstream. When the glucose level in the blood increases after a meal, the pancreas releases insulin into the bloodstream in response. Why is that important? Simply, insulin is required to transport glucose into all the body cells, where the glucose is used to produce energy. At the same time, insulin transports fat into the fat cells. So, while a fatty meal does not stimulate much insulin release, a carb meal stimulates a large release of insulin, which then transports glucose and any available fat in the blood into the fat cells for storage. Glucose, once inside the fat cells, is also converted to fat. On this basis, the role of insulin release in the genesis of the overweight and obese conditions cannot be overemphasized.

ALL CARBOHYDRATES ARE NOT CREATED EQUAL. Some carbs are quickly and easily converted to glucose while others are converted to glucose slowly and gradually. The former are said to have a high glycemic index (GI) or glycemic load (GL), and the latter are said to have a low GI or GL. The high GI carbs stimulate a much quicker and larger insulin release, leading to the production of stored fat in the fat cells much more easily than low GI carbs. Therefore, high GI (GL) is bad, and low GI (GL) is good, at least in terms of dealing with the overweight condition.

Because glycemic load also reflects the caloric density of food (the calories in a given amount of a particular food), GL is a better marker of good and bad carbs, and should be used to choose which foods to consume. The lower the GL, the better the carb is for you. A GL less than 10 is considered low, a GL between 10 and 19 is considered moderate, and a GL greater than 19 is high. High GL foods should be avoided as much as possible, moderate GL foods should be consumed in moderation, and low GL foods can be eaten liberally. Table 1 (Appendix 3) lists examples of various carbs and their GL.

2. FATS

Fat is stored in all the tissues of the body in the form of triglycerides (a combination of glycerol and fatty acids) and serves as an efficient source of stored energy. While some fat storage is necessary and healthy, excess fat storage is unhealthy.

.

Fat in the diet consists primarily of triglycerides and cholesterol. Fat from animal sources is primarily <u>SATURATED FAT,</u> which is unhealthy and is a major contributor to heart and circulatory disease. Fat from plant sources is primarily <u>UNSATURATED FAT</u> and actually leads to improved heart and circulatory health. These fats are digested and absorbed into the bloodstream in the small intestine, and then reconstituted. The triglycerides are then stored in fat cells unless they are utilized for energy immediately after they are absorbed, while cholesterol is used in many bodily functions including the production of cell membranes and the production of numerous hormones. Triglycerides serve as THE MAJOR CONTRIBUTOR to muscle metabolism, and therefore the lack of adequate exercise tends to increase the amount of stored fat in the body.

It cannot be overstated that INSULIN is required to store fat in the fat cells, and that GLUCOSE from carbs in the diet leads to insulin release, which leads to storage of fat in fat cells.

3. PROTEINS

Proteins are the "building blocks" of the body, and are the structural basis for muscle, connective tissue, and all enzymes. They are used for energy production by the body only as a last resort during conditions such as starvation. Muscle proteins play an important role in preventing overweight because of their role in physical exercise.

Exercise, if properly performed, can burn energy using carbs and fat before they can be converted to fat in fat cells. This is important because once fat is stored in fat cells, even more exercise is required to remove it than would have been required to prevent its storage in the first place. Exercise also tends to produce more muscle tissue, and a higher muscle mass has been show to increase the resting metabolism. This can play a major role in using carbs and fats for energy before they can be incorporated into fat cells.

4. VITAMINS AND MINERALS

Vitamins and minerals help the body to efficiently utilize carbs, fats, and proteins. They also are necessary for proper functioning of the various cells of the body. A nutritionally balanced diet generally provides all the vitamins and minerals required for good health, but during efforts at weight loss, there is a risk that the diet alone may not provide the necessary vitamins and minerals. For that reason, a multiple vitamin supplement is generally recommended as a component of the weight loss regimen. Additional supplementation with calcium, vitamin D, vitamin E, and "fish oil" (omega-3 fatty acids) may also be advisable. Your physician should be consulted regarding the appropriate use of supplements, especially those which are "out of the mainstream", such as megavitamins.

5. WATER

Healthy water intake varies according to daily activities. The more water that is lost, such as from the skin by sweating, and from the lungs during breathing, the more that needs to be replaced by drinking.

The typical 8-8 ounce glasses of water a day is a good general guideline but more is required as physical activity increases.

During weight loss, fat, and some protein, are broken down and eliminated from the body through the kidneys and liver as waste products. These waste products tend to carry extra water with them (into the urine, primarily), a process called diuresis. If extra water is not consumed during weight loss, dehydration can result. In addition, water helps prevent constipation. For these reasons, drinking lots of water during a weight-loss program is highly recommended.

6. FIBER

The portion of carbohydrates that is not digested and absorbed into the body is called fiber, and along with water forms the feces. Lots of fiber is important for healthy bowel function, and also helps prevent many diseases, such as diverticulosis, hemorrhoids, colon cancer, and diabetes. Remember, foods with a low glycemic load tend to be high in fiber, so structure your diet accordingly (see Appendix Table 2).

VII

The Importance Of "Nutrient Timing"

Based on the concepts of the Circadian rhythm of hormone release (especially cortisol) and the pre-eminent role of insulin in fat production, a rational theory of weight management can be proposed.

Cortisol tends to break down fat in the fat cells and release them into the bloodstream for use as an energy source. It stands to reason that during the morning and afternoon hours, when cortisol levels are relatively high, the fat cells are vulnerable to lose fat, especially if the person is physically active. On the other hand, at night, when cortisol levels are lower, fat is more easily incorporated into fat cells. If large amounts of insulin are available at this time, released by evening time consumption of high GI (GL) foods, the tendency to incorporate fat into fat cells is further increased. Finally, if the person is typically sleeping in the evening, and, therefore, inactive, the production of fat is further enhanced.

The essence of Circadian-based weight management is therefore:

1. Eat most of your calories before 4PM.
2. Eat a substantial breakfast.
3. Eat most of your carbs (especially high GI carbs) before 4PM, and
4. Minimize calories and carbs at the evening meal.

VIII

The Role Of Exercise

The benefits of regular exercise are widely known, both for general health and cardiovascular fitness, and for control of body weight. The explosion of obesity in the United States is due in large part to our sedentary lifestyle. Even modest amounts of physical activity incorporated into our daily lives can make a profound difference in our efforts toward good health and a healthy body weight. It's not necessary to be a marathon runner or world-class athlete to accomplish those goals.

What is adequate exercise? What types of exercise should I do? Those questions are frequently asked by people seeking to modify their lifestyles to improve their health. For most people, a combination of aerobic exercise (exercise which is maintained within the body's capacity to provide oxygen to the muscles on a sustained basis), and moderate strength training is all that is required. Often, this can be easily adapted to our daily schedules. IT IS WISE TO CONSULT WITH YOUR PHYSICIAN BEFORE EMBARKING ON A VIGOROUS EXERCISE PROGRAM.

It was previously thought that aerobic exercise had to be sustained for at least 20 minutes in order to be beneficial. Now it is known that aerobic exercise in increments as short as 5 to 10 minutes can be very beneficial. This fact allows flexibility in the incorporation of aerobic exercise into a daily routine. For example, take the stairs instead of the elevator. More examples will be given in Chapter IX.

1. Aerobic Exercise

    Common aerobic exercises include fast walking, jogging, running, bicycling, stair climbing, swimming, and cross-country skiing. Any exercise that allows sustained aerobic activity would qualify. How can you tell if you are exercising aerobically? Probably the best way is to measure your pulse. If you are not taking any medication that would slow your heart rate down, a pulse rate (number of beats per minute) between 2/3 and 3/4 of your maximum predicted heart (pulse) rate is in the aerobic range. What is the maximum predicted heart rate (MHR)? It is easily calculated as 220 minus your age in years. If you are 40 years old, MHR = 220-40, or 180. Your aerobic range is therefore a pulse rate between 120 (2/3 of 180) and 135 (3/4 of 180). Another good guideline is that if you cannot carry on a conversation with another person while exercising, you are probably exceeding the aerobic range (heart rate greater than MHR). Thirty minutes of aerobic exercise 3 or 4 times a week is adequate to achieve the desired results of good cardiovascular health and healthy weight maintenance. (Be sure to adequately stretch your muscles before each exercise session to help prevent injury).

2. Strengthening Exercise

Strength training using some type of resistance apparatus such as free weights or a weight machine can increase the body's muscle mass without producing much extra bulk. This extra muscle mass increases the resting metabolism, and allows the body to use up stored fat to provide that resting energy requirement, even when you're asleep! This benefit requires about 6 months after starting the exercise program to become apparent, so patience is a must. Before starting a strength-training program, seek professional advice from a trainer, if possible, to ensure proper technique and to help prevent injury.

IX.

Behavior Modification

There are many ways our daily activities can be quickly and simply altered to enhance the results of any weight management program. Individual creativity is the essence of each person's program, but there are some behavioral changes that are known to work for most people, and a number of these will be listed below. Entire books have been written on this subject and can be referenced by those who want to be more aggressive in this area. Keep in mind that changing behavior is not easy because we are creatures of habit, but the effort to change your habits is rewarded in the long run when the new behaviors themselves become habit and therefore automatic (this usually takes 3 to 6 months to establish).

1. Portion control – limit the size of each portion of food

on your plate to the size of the palm of your hand and NO SECONDS.

2. Eat your food in small bites and chew thoroughly before swallowing. Eating slowly enhances the enjoyment of the flavors of the food and allows the body to have time to say "enough".

3. Eat your meals at the table, preferably as a family or other group, and NOT IN FRONT OF THE TV. This allows healthy discourse and communication with others during the meal and promotes eating slowly.

4. Minimize time watching TV or other sedentary activity to no more than one-hour daily.

5. Eat a substantial breakfast daily.

6. Drink lots of water (at least eight 8 ounce glasses daily).

7. Limit fast foods to once a week.

8. Limit alcohol intake to one mixed drink or 4 ounces of wine daily.

9. Eliminate sugar from the diet; use artificial sweeteners instead.

10. Avoid foods with a high caloric density (lots of calories in a small amount of food), and fall in love with foods with a low caloric density, such as fruits, vegetables, and whole grains. Coincidentally, high GL foods and fat tend to have a high caloric density, and low GL foods tend to have a low caloric density.

11. Weigh yourself on the same scales weekly and RECORD your weight. The purpose of this is not

to focus on day-to-day variations, but to examine TRENDS in your weight over time.

12. Set realistic goals and expectations. If you weigh 350 pounds, don't expect to achieve a weight of 150 pounds in 6 months. Instead, focus on a more realistic objective of 325 pounds in 6-12 months, with a long-term goal of 200 pounds of body weight in 2 to 3 years, also allowing time for behavior change to become habit. Remember, unrealistic expectations are self-defeating.

13. Exercise whenever feasible, even in small increments. Take the stairs; park a distance from the building and walk instead of parking close to the building; walk quickly, not slowly; use lawn and garden activities as a source of exercise; walk around the block during your lunch hour; walk your dog or cat; and BE CREATIVE.

14. Read labels on food and drink. Educate yourself to know what you're eating.

15. Make it a group effort. If you have friends or family who also need weight management, start a group and do it together. Peer pressure works wonders to help realize change in behavior.

16. Keep a periodic diary of your food intake, particularly at the beginning of the weight management program, even if you are losing weight as expected or maintaining a healthy weight.

17. Finally, remember that TIME is your ally, so keep your focus on the long term, be patient, and keep your eyes on the prize – a pleasing appearance and good health.

X

Medical And Surgical Weight Loss

Morbid obesity is typically defined as a BMI greater than 40 (or greater than 35 for people with illnesses such as diabetes, high blood pressure, and heart disease). People with morbid obesity need to lose weight rapidly because of the high health risk of their obesity. Rapid weight loss techniques are risky themselves, but often the risk of obesity is greater. If you are morbidly obese, a consultation with your physician is recommended to determine if a more aggressive weight loss method is for you. Remember, these methods produce only short-term results, and still should be incorporated into a long-term weight management program.

What are the more aggressive methods?

1. Very-low-calorie diets. These are typically liquid prescription diets providing daily calories in the range of 400 to 800, requiring close medical supervision.

2. Medications. Many medications have been used for short-term weight loss. Some are more risky than others, but none are without risk. Humans are creatures of habit, and effective weight management requires changing from unhealthy habits to healthy habits. This process requires from 3 to 6 months, and weight loss medications can act as a "bridge" to enable weight loss while habits are being changed. Safer and more effective medications are being developed but are not yet available. Close medical supervision is required, and courses of treatment longer than 6 months are not currently recommended.

3. Surgery. Surgical procedures are reserved for the most severe and resistant cases of morbid obesity and should be considered a last resort. While the procedures are effective, there are potentially severe short and long term complications, and the long-term health consequences are not fully known. Surgery should not be undertaken lightly, and comprehensive pre-operative evaluation is required, including physical, nutritional, and psychological screening. Ideally, these procedures should be performed by a surgeon who specializes in this area of practice, allowing him/her to perform a high volume of procedures in the context of a comprehensive long-term weight management program.

DRASTIC SITUATIONS OFTEN CALL FOR DRASTIC MEASURES.

XI

Psychological Factors

When embarking upon a weight management program, be aware that psychological factors can impair your efforts, and can even indicate an underlying psychological illness. The trick is to turn psychology into your ally.

A. If you perceive yourself as overweight, but your BMI is normal or even low, you may have an eating disorder such as anorexia nervosa or bulimia. In this case, consultation with a physician is advisable.

B. If you eat excessively in response to life stressors, such as job stress, financial problems, marital discord, etc., you may be a compulsive overeater. Consultation with a physician or psychologist is advisable.

C. Be aware that "significant others" occasionally sabotage the weight management efforts of their loved ones if they perceive the weight loss as a threat to the relationship.

For example, if both spouses are overweight, and one spouse embarks upon a weight loss program, the second spouse may feel threatened as the first spouse loses weight and becomes "more physically attractive" to others. The second spouse may combat the circumstance by tempting the first spouse to eat more, thereby sabotaging the weight loss effort.

D. Humans are creatures of habit. Long-term weight management requires lifestyle change, which means substituting "good (healthy)" habits for "bad (unhealthy)" ones. Studies have demonstrated that 3 to 6 months are required to effect a habit change, and to maintain the newly developed good habit requires a brief reminder every 3 to 6 months. For example, once a healthy weight is achieved, a periodic review of healthy eating and exercise habits helps to maintain and reinforce those habits. Healthy weight maintenance is indeed a lifetime project, which also "prolongs the lifetime". This is well worth the effort.

XII

The Final Story:
Another Inconvenient Truth

There is an old, humorous saying that *when all is said and done, more is said than done.* Unfortunately, that applies to most of our efforts to effectively manage our body weight in a healthy fashion. I am convinced that we can do better. All it takes is knowledge and commitment. Hopefully, this book will provide you with the knowledge you need to manage your weight, and the motivation to commit to a plan to achieve your goal – maintaining your weight in a healthy range.

The energy you consume in the form of food and drink, minus the energy that your body utilizes in your daily activities determines whether you gain weight (store fat), lose weight (eliminate fat), or maintain your present weight. Since the calorie is a measure of energy, if you consume more calories than you expend, you will gain weight in the form of fat (stored energy).

If you consume fewer calories than you expend, you will lose weight – preferably fat and not muscle tissue if you minimize bad carbs and fat in the diet and exercise to build and strengthen muscle.

The Delta Diet concept, if properly and faithfully executed, can help you to use the calories you consume only to perform your daily activities rather than store excess calories as fat. But, there is no magic, and no way to circumvent the laws of nature. If you do not consume fewer calories than you burn every day, you WILL NOT lose weight consistently. That is the final, though sometimes, inconvenient truth.

Good luck as you implement the specific steps recommended in Appendices 1 & 2 of this book.

APPENDICES

Appendix 1

General Guidelines For Food Intake

The following general guidelines are a good starting point regarding daily food intake. Specific diet plans will be offered in Appendix 5.

1. Total daily calories to maintain your weight can be calculated as follows:

    For men: [900 + 4.55 x (wt in pounds)] x Activity Factor (AF)

    For women: [700 + 3.18 x (wt in pounds)] x Activity Factor (AF)

    For Sedentary Lifestyle: AF = 1.3

    For Average Lifestyle: AF = 1.5

    For example, a woman who weighs 130 pounds and gets minimal exercise should eat no more than [700 + 3.18 x 130], or

1467 calories per day to maintain her weight. To lose weight, she would have to either eat less, exercise more, or a combination of both. On average, reducing the weight maintenance calories by 500 each day would produce a weight loss of 1 pound per week.

2. Nutrients
    a. Eat lots of protein (25-30% of total calories)
    b. Eat lots of low GI carbs and very few high GI carbs (total carbs about 50-55% of total calories).
    c. Eat SOME fat (20-25% of total calories). Most of the fat should come from plant sources, which is mostly unsaturated, and not animal sources, which is mostly saturated.
    d. Drink lots of water
3. Timing
    a. Eat 70-80% of calories before 6 PM (adjust the time if you are on shift work).
4. Healthy Habits
    a. Whole foods (unprocessed foods) are better than processed foods.
    b. Fresh foods are best, with frozen foods being a close second. Canned foods, as a general rule, are best avoided because they tend to have more additives, including lots of sodium. READ THE LABELS BEFORE CONSUMING.
    c. Eliminate sugar, potatoes, white rice, and any food incorporating white flour from the diet.
    d. Eliminate any food with a glycemic load greater than 19 from the diet.
    e. Portion control is important. Each portion of food should be no larger than the palm of your hand, and NO SECONDS!
    f. Keep a periodic diary of your food intake. This is especially important at the beginning of the

weight management program, and during weight maintenance (every 1-3 months).

APPENDIX 2

The 1,2,3 Of The Delta Diet

(COPY THIS PAGE AND PLACE ON YOUR REFRIGERATOR DOOR)

It's as easy as:

1. Avoid food after 6 PM. Eat no more than 20% of your calories after 6 PM.

2. Avoid "bad" carbohydrates and saturated fats. "Bad" carbohydrates include sugar, white bread or anything else made with white flour, potatoes, and white rice. Saturated fats include lard, shortening, and butter. Especially bad are combinations of "bad" carbohydrates and fat, such as French fries, potato chips, and donuts.

3. Encourage fresh fruits and vegetables, unprocessed cereals

and other whole grains. Also lean meats, chicken, and fish (preferably baked, broiled, sautéed, or grilled).
Also,

4.   AVOID FAST FOODS AND SOFT DRINKS

5.   Limit portions size to no larger than the palm of your hand, and keep a DIET DIARY

(Moderate exercise, such as walking, is recommended to enhance the effect of the diet. Be creative. For instance, take the stairs instead of the elevator, park the car across the parking lot from the store and walk, and walk in the airport while waiting for your flight).

Make your motto: WALK FAST, EAT SLOWLY!!!!

APPENDIX 3

Table 1
Glycemic Load Chart

Food	Serving	Glycemic Load per Serving	Category Lower is Better
Bakery Products & Bread			

Food	Serving	Glycemic Load per Serving	Category Lower is Better
Banana Cake (made with sugar)	3	18	medium
Banana Cake (made without sugar)	3	16	medium

Sponge Cake, plain	2	17	medium
Vanilla Cake made from packet mix with vanilla frosting (Betty Crocker)	4	111	high
Apple Pie (made with sugar)	2	13	medium
Apple Pie (made without sugar)	2	9	low
Waffles, Aunt Jemima	1	10	low
Bagel, white frozen	3	25	high
Baguette, white, plain	1	15	medium
Coarse barley bread	1	7	low
Hamburger bun	1	9	low
Kaiser bun	1	12	medium
Pumpernickel bread	1	6	low
50% cracked wheat bread	1	12	medium
White wheat flour bread	1	10	low
Wonder bread	1	10	low
Whole-wheat bread	1	9	low
100% whole grain bread	1	7	low
Pita bread, white	1	10	low

Corn tortilla	2	12	medium
Wheat tortilla	2	8	low

Beverages

Coca Cola	9	15	Medium
Fanta	9	23	high
Lucozade	9	40	high
Apple Juice	9	12	medium
Cranberry Juice	9	24	high
Grapefruit Juice	9	11	medium
Orange Juice	9	13	medium
Tomato Juice	9	4	low

Grains

Pearled barley	5	11	medium
Sweet corn on the cob	5	17	
Couscous	5	23	high
White rice	5	23	high
Brown rice	5	18	medium

Breakfast			
All-bran	1	4	low
Coco Pops	1	20	high
Cornflakes	9	21	high
Cream of Wheat	9	17	medium
Grapenuts	1	22	high
Muesli	1	15	medium
Oatmeal	9	16	medium
Instant Oatmeal	9	13	medium
Puffed Wheat	1	17	medium
Raisin Bran	1	16	medium
Special K	1	12	medium

Cookies and Crackers			
Graham Crackers	2	14	medium
Vanilla Wafers	2	14	medium
Shortbread	2	10	low

Rice Cakes	2	17	medium
Rye Crisps	2	11	medium
Soda Crackers	2	12	medium

Daily Products & Alternatives			

Ice Cream	2	8	low
Milk, full fat	9	4	low
Milk, skim	9	3	low
Reduced-fat yogurt with fruit	7	4	low

Fruit			

Apple	4	6	low
Banana	2	13	medium
Dates	4	42	High
Grapefruit	4	3	low
Grapes	4	8	low
Orange	4	5	low
Peach	4	5	low

Pear	4	9	low
Prunes	4	4	low
Raisins	2	5	low
Watermelon	2	10	low

Beans and Nuts			

Baked Beans	5	7	low
Black Beans	5	13	medium
Chickpeas	5	7	low
Navy Beans	5	8	low
Kidney Beans	5	9	low
Lentils	5	12	medium
Soy Beans	5	7	low
Almonds	2	1	low
Cashews	2	5	low
Peanuts	2	1	low

Pasta and Noodles			

Fettuccini	6	18	medium
Macaroni	6	23	high
Macaroni and Cheese (Kraft)	6	32	high
Spaghetti	6	18	medium

Snack Food			

Corn Chips	1	17	medium
Fruit Roll-Ups	1	24	high
M&M's	1	6	low
Microwave Popcorn	2	8	low
Potato Chips	1	11	Medium
Pretzels	2	16	medium
Snicker Bar	2	19	medium
Green Peas	3	3	low
Carrots	3	3	low
Parsnips	5	12	medium
White Potato	5	26	high

Sweet Potato	5	14	medium
Yam	5	17	medium
Hummus	1	0	low
Chicken Nuggets	4	7	low
Pizza (Cheese & Sauce)	4	22	high
Pizza Supreme	4	9	low
Honey	1	10	low

APPENDIX 4

BMI Table

Healthy Weight

Being overweight can elevate your blood pressure, lead to Type 2 diabetes, and increase your risk for heart disease, cancer, arthritis, and depression. Body Mass Index (BMI) is the most common measure for defining if you are overweight or obese. It accounts for both height and weight.

Risk Level	BMI
Healthy Weight	18.5 to 24.9
Overweight	25 to 29.9
Obese	30 to 39.9
Morbidly Obese	40

Body Mass Index (BMI)

Weight In Pounds

BMI	19	20	21	22	23	24	25	26	27	28	29	30	35	40
Height in Inches														
58	91	96	100	105	110	115	119	124	129	134	138	143	167	191
59	94	99	104	109	114	119	124	128	133	138	143	148	173	198
60	97	102	107	112	118	123	133	137	143	148	153	159	179	204
61	100	106	111	116	122	127	132	138	143	148	153	159	185	211
62	104	109	115	120	126	131	136	142	147	153	158	164	191	218
63	107	113	118	124	130	135	141	146	152	158	163	169	197	225
64	110	116	122	128	134	140	145	151	157	163	169	174	204	232
65	114	120	126	132	138	144	150	156	162	168	174	180	210	240
66	118	124	130	136	142	148	155	161	167	173	179	186	216	247
67	121	127	134	140	146	153	159	166	172	178	185	191	223	255
68	125	131	138	144	151	158	164	171	177	184	190	197	230	262
69	128	135	142	149	155	162	169	176	182	189	196	203	236	270
70	132	139	146	153	160	157	174	181	188	195	202	207	243	278
71	136	143	150	157	165	172	179	186	193	200	208	215	250	286
72	140	147	154	162	169	177	184	191	199	206	213	221	258	294
73	144	151	159	166	174	182	189	197	204	212	219	227	265	302
74	148	155	163	171	179	186	194	202	210	218	225	233	272	311
75	152	160	168	176	184	192	200	208	216	224	232	240	279	319
76	156	164	172	180	189	197	205	213	221	230	238	246	287	328
	Healthy						Overweight						Obese	

APPENDIX 5

SAMPLE MENUS

<u>1200 Calorie per Day Diet</u>

Meal Plan 1

<u>Breakfast</u>
1 Cup Fruit Juice
½ Cup Oatmeal
1 Cup Low-Fat Yogurt
Black Coffee or Herbal Tea

<u>Snack</u>
Smoothie
(1 cup berries blended with 1 cup Trim (1%) milk and ice cubes)

<u>Lunch</u>
2 Slices Whole Wheat Bread
½ Cup Tuna (in water only)
Salad (Tomato, Cucumber, Lettuce) with 1 teaspoon mayonnaise + ½ tbsp olive oil)

<u>Dinner</u>
3.5 oz (~100g) Chicken Breast (skinless, boneless) – cook in griller
1 Cup Broccoli
½ Cup Brown Rice

Meal Plan 2

Breakfast
2 Slices Whole Wheat Toast with 1 tsp Butter
½ Cup Canned Fruit Cocktail (fruit salad) – in natural juice ONLY
8 oz (1 cup) Trim (1%) Milk

Snack
1 Medium-Sized Banana

Lunch
6 Crackers with Low-Fat Cottage Cheese
Handful Mixed Nuts (Almonds, Walnuts, Brazilian Nuts)
1 Medium Fruit (Apple, Peach, Plum, Pear, etc.)

Dinner
Medium Baked Potato
3 oz (~85g) Sirloin Steak
½ Cup Mushrooms
¼ Cup Onions
1 Teaspoon Olive or Canola Oil (cooking)
1 Cup Mixed Vegetables

1400 Calorie per Day Diet

Meal Plan 1

Breakfast
1 Cup Cantaloupe
Scrambled Eggs (1/2 cup egg substitute or 1 egg and 1 egg white, 1 tsp butter)
English muffin (dry, whole wheat)

Snack
Mug of Granola (2 tablespoon granola + ¼ cup fat-free milk)

Lunch
1 Cup Fat-Free Milk
Peanut Butter and Jelly Sandwich (2 tbsp peanut butter, 2 tbsp jelly or jam, 2 slices whole wheat bread)
½ Cup Celery Sticks and ½ Cup Baby Carrots

Dinner
Mixes Greens (2 cups + 1 tbsp reduced-calorie dressing)
Spaghetti (1 cup whole wheat spaghetti, ¼ cup meatless pasta sauce, 2 tbsp Parmesan Cheese, 2 teaspoons chopped basil)

Treat
3 Ginger Snaps

Meal Plan 2

Breakfast
1 Cup Fat-Free Milk
½ Cup Strawberries
English Muffin (with butter and jam) – Whole Wheat or Oat bran + 1 teaspoon butter

Snack
1 Graham Cracker
1 Cup Chocolate Milk
Fat-Free Milk + 2 tbsp
Chocolate Syrup

Lunch
Small Roll – 2 ½ inches in size
Veggie Salad – (1 cup mixed greens, 1/3 cup carrots, 1/3 cup tomatoes, 1/3 cup cucumbers, ½ cup canned chickpeas, 2 tbsp chopped egg, 2 tbsp reduced-calorie dressing)

Dinner
4 oz Whole Wheat Spaghetti or 2 Cups Ziti
2 Cups Broccoli Florets (coarsely chopped)
1 Cup Sliced, Cooked Chicken Breast
4 tbsp grated Parmesan Cheese
4 teaspoons Olive Oil
Pinch of Red Pepper (optional)
- Prepare the pasta according to package directions. Drain, reserving 1 cup of the liquid. Return the liquid to the pot. Place the pasta in a bowl and cover to keep warm. Bring the liquid to a boil. Add the broccoli, cover and cook for 4 to 5 minutes, or until soft but not soggy. Add the pasta, chicken, cheese, oil, and pepper flakes (if using). Toss well and enjoy!

Treat

Frozen Fruit Bar – no more than 80 Calories

<u>1600 Calorie per Day Diet</u>

Meal Plan 1

<u>Breakfast</u>
1 Cup Fat-Free Milk
2 Whole Grain Toaster Waffles, topped with one of the following:

>1 Cup Berries
>2 tsp Butter or Trans-Free Margarine
>2 tsp Maple Syrup

<u>Morning Snack</u>
2 tsp Peanut Butter
2 Graham Crackers
Maple Milk (1 cup fat-free milk + 1 tsp maple syrup)

<u>Lunch</u>
1 Cup sliced Red Peppers
Veggie Cheeseburger

>1 Vegetable burger (such as Garden Burger)
>1 slice Reduced-Fat Cheese
>1 Whole Wheat hamburger bun
>2 tsp Low-Fat Mayo and Mustard
>2 Tomato slices
>2 pieces of Lettuce
>Cook 1 Vegetable Burger according to package directions.

Melt 1 slice reduced-fat cheese on top and place 1 whole wheat hamburger bun with 2 tsp low-fat mayo, mustard, tomato slices, and lettuce.

<u>Afternoon Snack</u>
1 Protein Bar (20g protein)

Dinner

1 Cup steamed Broccoli, with sprits of Lemon Juice

Lemon Couscous

    2/3 cup of Water

    ½ tsp of Butter

    Dash of Salt

    ⅓ cup of Dry, Whole Wheat Couscous

    2 tbsp Raisins

    1 tsp grated Lemon Zest

    Cook: In a small saucepan, bring water, butter, and salt to a boil. Add the

Couscous. Cover, turn off heat, and let stand for 5 minutes. Fluff with a fork. Add the raisins and lemon zest. Toss to combine.

Fish with Olive and Capers

    2 tsp of Olive Oil

    1 clove of Garlic (chopped)

    1 14oz can whole Tomato Peppers

    2 Fish fillets (red snapper, tilapia, or other fish, 5-6 oz each)

    2 ½ tbsp chopped, fresh basil

    2 tbsp chopped and pitted Black Olives

    1 tsp chopped Capers

    Cook: In a large, nonstick skillet, warm the oil over medium heat. Add the garlic and stir for 30 seconds. Add the tomatoes. Bring to a boil, breaking the tomatoes into coarse chunks with a spoon. Reduce the heat to medium-low and simmer for 10 minutes, season with pepper. Add the fish and spoon the sauce over it to cover completely. Cover and simmer for 10 minutes or until fish flakes easily. Transfer just the fish to a serving dish. Stir basil, olives, and capers into the tomatoes. Simmer for 30 seconds and pour over the fish.

<u>Treat</u>
5 Chips Ahoy! Cookies

Meal Plan 2

Breakfast
Cereal
1 cup Fat-Free Milk
1 small Banana, sliced

Morning Snack
2 tbsp Almonds
8 oz/226g Low-Fat Fruit Yogurt with no more than 210 calories
2 tsp Peanut Butter

Lunch
1 Orange
½ cup Low-Fat Cottage Cheese
1 cup sliced Red Peppers
Turkey and Cheese Sandwich
    2 slices Whole Wheat Bread
    2 slices Turkey Breast
    2 slices Reduced-Fat Cheese
    2 Tomato slices
    1 Leaf Lettuce
    1 tsp Low-Fat Mayo
    1 tsp Mustard

Dinner
1 cup Brown Rice
Shrimp and Vegetable Kabobs
    6 oz raw shrimp (about 14 shrimp)
    2 peeled medium onions cut into wedges
    1 cup small, whole mushrooms or Portabella mushrooms cut into large wedges
    2/3 cup cherry tomatoes

Juice of 1 lemon

1 tablespoon olive oil

1 clove garlic

Crushed salt and pepper to taste

2 tablespoons chopped fresh dill, parsley, or basil (optional)

Cook: If using wooden skewers, soak them in cold water for about 10 minutes. Preheat the broiler or an outdoor grill. Alternate the shrimp and about half the onions on 2 skewers. Alternate the mushrooms, tomatoes, and remaining onions on 2 skewers. In a small bowl, mix the lemon juice, oil, and garlic or garlic powder. Pour half into a cup and set aside. Brush the remainder over the skewers and discard any that's left. Place the vegetable skewers on a broiler pan or outdoor grill. Broil or grill for about 2 minutes per side. Add the shrimp skewers. Cook for 5-7 minutes, turning all the skewers after about 3 minutes. Using a clean brush, brush the skewers with the reserved lemon mixture. (A clean brush prevents possible contamination with bacteria from raw shrimp on the first brush). Season with salt and pepper. Sprinkle with herbs (if using).

Treat

2 Keebler Sandies Cookies

Ensure you drink plenty of water – aim for 8-10 glasses per day!

APPENDIX 6

Protein Supplements

Protein supplements (snacks), such as bars and shakes, are useful to help ensure that you are losing fat, not protein, during your weight loss efforts. Protein is the major component of muscle, including the heart, and protein malnutrition can lead to serious medical complications. In addition, loss of muscle mass can impair physical fitness and hence the ability to maintain an adequate exercise program.

Acceptable protein supplements should provide no more than 150 calories per serving, mostly protein, with only enough carbohydrate for flavoring and enough fat to bind the product together. As a bonus, these products tend to be quite filling, eliminating that between-meal "hunger pangs". Convenient packaging to ensure portability and flexibility of use is a must. The snack must be available when needed.

The following page lists the nutritional composition of

some acceptable protein supplements, and may be helpful for comparison-shopping.

Acceptable Nutritional Content for Protein Bars

Serving Size	40g	40b	40g	40g	40g
Calories	150	150	150	150	160
Total Fat	3g	3g	3g	2.5g	2.5g
Saturated Fat	1g	0g	1g	0g	0g
Trans Fat	0g	0g	0g	0g	0g
Cholesterol	0mg	0mg	0mg	0mg	0mg
Sodium	200mg	200mg	180mg	135mg	85mg
Potassium	50mg	50mg	55mg	25mg	35mg
Total Carbohydrate	20gg	20g	21g	22g	30g
Fiber (Soluble)	6g	5g	5g	6g	<1g
Sugar	0g	0g	0g	1g	10g
Sugar Alcohol	4g	6g	6g	5g	5g
Protein	12g	12g	11g	12g	4g
Calcium	4% DV	4% DV	4% DV	4% DV	2% DV
Iron	10% DV	10% DV	10% DV	10% DV	4% DV
Phorphorous	10% DV	10% DV	10% DV	10% DV	2% DV
Glycemic Index	41	32	33	42	51
Glycemic Load	5	4	4	12	14

DV = Daily Value

Daily Food Diary - Date: _____

Time	Food of Drink	Serving Size	Hunger Level 1 = Starving, 5 = Full	Mood	Alone or With Others	Where

Drank Water ☐ ☐ ☐ ☐ ☐ ☐ ☐ ☐

Multi-Vitamin ☐

Exercise _____

Daily Food Diary - Date: _____

Time	Food of Drink	Serving Size	Hunger Level 1= Starving, 5= Full	Mood	Alone or With Others	Where

Drank Water ☐ ☐ ☐ ☐ ☐ ☐ ☐ ☐
Multi-Vitamin ☐
Exercise _____

Daily Food Diary - Date: _____

Time	Food of Drink	Serving Size	Hunger Level 1= Starving, 5= Full	Mood	Alone or With Others	Where

Drank Water ☐ ☐ ☐ ☐ ☐ ☐ ☐ ☐

Multi-Vitamin ☐

Exercise _____

Daily Food Diary - Date: _____

Time	Food of Drink	Serving Size	Hunger Level 1= Starving, 5= Full	Mood	Alone or With Others	Where

Drank Water ☐ ☐ ☐ ☐ ☐ ☐ ☐ ☐
Multi-Vitamin ☐
Exercise _____

Daily Food Diary - Date: _____

Time	Food of Drink	Serving Size	Hunger Level 1 = Starving, 5 = Full	Mood	Alone or With Others	Where

Drank Water ☐ ☐ ☐ ☐ ☐ ☐ ☐ ☐
Multi-Vitamin ☐
Exercise _____

Daily Food Diary - Date: _____

Time	Food of Drink	Serving Size	Hunger Level 1 = Starving, 5 = Full	Mood	Alone or With Others	Where

Drank Water ☐ ☐ ☐ ☐ ☐ ☐ ☐ ☐

Multi-Vitamin ☐

Exercise _____

Daily Food Diary - Date: _____

Time	Food of Drink	Serving Size	Hunger Level 1 = Starving, 5 = Full	Mood	Alone or With Others	Where

Drank Water ☐ ☐ ☐ ☐ ☐ ☐ ☐ ☐

Multi-Vitamin ☐

Exercise _____

Daily Food Diary - Date: _____

Time	Food of Drink	Serving Size	Hunger Level 1 = Starving, 5 = Full	Mood	Alone or With Others	Where

Drank Water ☐ ☐ ☐ ☐ ☐ ☐

Multi-Vitamin ☐

Exercise _____

Daily Food Diary - Date: _____

Time	Food of Drink	Serving Size	Hunger Level 1 = Starving, 5= Full	Mood	Alone or With Others	Where

Drank Water ☐ ☐ ☐ ☐ ☐ ☐ ☐
Multi-Vitamin ☐
Exercise _____

Daily Food Diary - Date: _____

Time	Food of Drink	Serving Size	Hunger Level 1 = Starving, 5 = Full	Mood	Alone or With Others	Where

Drank Water ☐ ☐ ☐ ☐ ☐ ☐ ☐
Multi-Vitamin ☐
Exercise _____

Daily Food Diary - Date: _____

Time	Food of Drink	Serving Size	Hunger Level 1 = Starving, 5 = Full	Mood	Alone or With Others	Where

Drank Water ☐ ☐ ☐ ☐ ☐ ☐ ☐ ☐
Multi-Vitamin ☐
Exercise _____

Daily Food Diary - Date: _____

Time	Food of Drink	Serving Size	Hunger Level 1= Starving, 5= Full	Mood	Alone or With Others	Where

Drank Water ☐ ☐ ☐ ☐ ☐ ☐ ☐ ☐
Multi-Vitamin ☐
Exercise _____

Daily Food Diary - Date: _____

Time	Food of Drink	Serving Size	Hunger Level 1= Starving, 5= Full	Mood	Alone or With Others	Where

Drank Water ☐ ☐ ☐ ☐ ☐ ☐ ☐ ☐
Multi-Vitamin ☐
Exercise _____

Daily Food Diary - Date: _____

Time	Food of Drink	Serving Size	Hunger Level 1= Starving, 5= Full	Mood	Alone or With Others	Where

Drank Water ☐ ☐ ☐ ☐ ☐ ☐ ☐ ☐
Multi-Vitamin ☐
Exercise _____

Daily Food Diary - Date: _____

Time	Food of Drink	Serving Size	Hunger Level 1= Starving, 5= Full	Mood	Alone or With Others	Where

Drank Water ☐ ☐ ☐ ☐ ☐ ☐ ☐ ☐

Multi-Vitamin ☐

Exercise _____

Daily Food Diary - Date: _____

Time	Food of Drink	Serving Size	Hunger Level 1 = Starving, 5 = Full	Mood	Alone or With Others	Where

Drank Water ☐ ☐ ☐ ☐ ☐ ☐ ☐ ☐
Multi-Vitamin ☐
Exercise _____

Daily Food Diary - Date: _____

Time	Food of Drink	Serving Size	Hunger Level 1 = Starving, 5 = Full	Mood	Alone or With Others	Where

Drank Water ☐ ☐ ☐ ☐ ☐ ☐ ☐ ☐

Multi-Vitamin ☐

Exercise _____

Daily Food Diary - Date: _____

Time	Food of Drink	Serving Size	Hunger Level 1 = Starving, 5= Full	Mood	Alone or With Others	Where

Drank Water ☐ ☐ ☐ ☐ ☐ ☐ ☐
Multi-Vitamin ☐
Exercise _____

Daily Food Diary - Date: _____

Time	Food of Drink	Serving Size	Hunger Level 1 = Starving, 5 = Full	Mood	Alone or With Others	Where

Drank Water ☐ ☐ ☐ ☐ ☐ ☐ ☐ ☐
Multi-Vitamin ☐
Exercise _____

Daily Food Diary - Date: _____

Time	Food of Drink	Serving Size	Hunger Level 1= Starving, 5= Full	Mood	Alone or With Others	Where

Drank Water ☐ ☐ ☐ ☐ ☐ ☐ ☐ ☐

Multi-Vitamin ☐

Exercise _____

Daily Food Diary - Date: _____

Time	Food of Drink	Serving Size	Hunger Level 1 = Starving, 5 = Full	Mood	Alone or With Others	Where

Drank Water ☐ ☐ ☐ ☐ ☐ ☐ ☐ ☐
Multi-Vitamin ☐
Exercise _____

Daily Food Diary - Date: _____

Time	Food of Drink	Serving Size	Hunger Level 1= Starving, 5= Full	Mood	Alone or With Others	Where

Drank Water ☐ ☐ ☐ ☐ ☐ ☐ ☐
Multi-Vitamin ☐
Exercise _____

Daily Food Diary - Date: _____

Time	Food of Drink	Serving Size	Hunger Level 1 = Starving, 5 = Full	Mood	Alone or With Others	Where

Drank Water ☐ ☐ ☐ ☐ ☐ ☐ ☐ ☐

Multi-Vitamin ☐

Exercise _____

Daily Food Diary - Date: _____

Time	Food of Drink	Serving Size	Hunger Level 1= Starving, 5= Full	Mood	Alone or With Others	Where

Drank Water ☐ ☐ ☐ ☐ ☐ ☐ ☐ ☐

Multi-Vitamin ☐

Exercise _____

Daily Food Diary - Date: _____

Time	Food of Drink	Serving Size	Hunger Level 1 = Starving, 5 = Full	Mood	Alone or With Others	Where

Drank Water ☐ ☐ ☐ ☐ ☐ ☐ ☐ ☐

Multi-Vitamin ☐

Exercise _____

Daily Food Diary - Date: _____

Time	Food of Drink	Serving Size	Hunger Level 1 = Starving, 5 = Full	Mood	Alone or With Others	Where

Drank Water ☐ ☐ ☐ ☐ ☐ ☐ ☐ ☐
Multi-Vitamin ☐
Exercise _____

Daily Food Diary - Date: _____

Time	Food of Drink	Serving Size	Hunger Level 1 = Starving, 5 = Full	Mood	Alone or With Others	Where

Drank Water ☐ ☐ ☐ ☐ ☐ ☐ ☐ ☐
Multi-Vitamin ☐
Exercise _____

Daily Food Diary - Date: _____

Time	Food of Drink	Serving Size	Hunger Level 1 = Starving, 5 = Full	Mood	Alone or With Others	Where

Drank Water ☐ ☐ ☐ ☐ ☐ ☐ ☐ ☐
Multi-Vitamin ☐
Exercise _____

Daily Food Diary - Date: _____

Time	Food of Drink	Serving Size	Hunger Level 1 = Starving, 5 = Full	Mood	Alone or With Others	Where

Drank Water ☐ ☐ ☐ ☐ ☐ ☐ ☐ ☐

Multi-Vitamin ☐

Exercise _____

Daily Food Diary - Date: _____

Time	Food of Drink	Serving Size	Hunger Level 1 = Starving, 5 = Full	Mood	Alone or With Others	Where

Drank Water ☐ ☐ ☐ ☐ ☐ ☐ ☐ ☐

Multi-Vitamin ☐

Exercise _____

About the Author

George E. Abraham II, MD, PHD, is a board-certified family physician who has practiced family medicine in Vicksburg, Mississippi since 1978. Dr. Abraham has a deep commitment to wellness and has integrated wellness and patient education into his practice. For his efforts, in 1989 he was honored with the _Patient Care_ award for Excellence in Patient Education. Dr. Abraham considers obesity a major health challenge for the U.S., and has written this book based on the information he shares with his patients in his daily practice of medicine.